Table of (

MW00562452

Jim's Weight Training & Bodybuilding Workout Plan

Build muscle and strength, burn fat & tone up with a full year of progressive weight training workouts

Jimshealthandmuscle.com

Copyright © 2013 by jimshealthandmuscle.com

Visit my blog for other great advice on diet, training, healthy recipes, motivation and more

www.jimshealthandmuscle.com

Please also "Like" at

www.facebook.com/jimshealthandmuscle

And Follow on Twitter

@jimshm

Preface

H i, I'm Jim, a qualified fitness coach with a thirst for helping people to reach their fitness potential.

During my time in the "fitness arena" I've been a long distance runner, competing bodybuilder and served a number of years in the British army in an airborne unit (9 para sqn R.E)

You will find out a lot more about me and a whole bunch of extra health, fitness and nutrition advice if you visit my website:

Jimshealthandmuscle.com

I'd like to thank you for your purchase and I know that you will get some great fitness results if you take on-board and act on the information that you read.

I always put a great focus on fitness results for the long term in my work and it is a "no brainer" to me that this approach is the best way to go with any fitness goal.

Before you start this training routine, please check out my author page as there may be other titles that will help you that out little bit more:

James Atkinson (author page)

I would also like to let you know that if you have any questions or comments, I would be more than happy to help you as these subjects are a passion of mine and have been for many years.

my mailing list & Free healthy recipes

———

If you would like to be notified of any future promotions, new releases or special offers that I have on health, fitness, diet and lifestyle please sign up to my mailing list

I promote every book on its release at $0.99 or even free of charge, and I would like to offer these opportunities to my loyal readers.

Why would I do this? First off, it is a "thank you" from me for choosing to buy my book over all of the competition

And secondly because I am a self-published author and I hold all the cards when it comes to promotion as well as writing the actual book, so the more hands that I can put my book into the better, and why shouldn't my existing customers be amongst this group of people?

Don't worry I hate spam emails too and I get my fair share so I rarely send out emails, but when I do, it will be something worth your while.

Please follow the link below to grab your 7 free healthy and tasty recipes that I have created myself. There are even pictures of the finished dishes that I have taken from my own kitchen so you know what to expect.

This free gift will help you out even more with your health and fitness plans and it also serves as a big thank you from me for your support.

Simply click this link or copy it into your browser and let me know where to send them!

https://jimshealthandmuscle.com/healthy-recipes-sign-up/

YOU MAY ALSO BE INTERESTED in my "Home Workout Series". Sometimes you just can't get to the gym, you are away on business or your gym is closed. Having a home workout plan to fall back on in these situations can be a great help!

Here is something that you can use for these circumstances:

HOME WORKOUT
CIRCUIT TRAINING

6 WEEK EXERCISE BAND WORKOUT & BODYWEIGHT
TRAINING FOR FAT LOSS, STRENGTH AND MUSCLE TONE

JAMES ATKINSON

Why I Wrote This Book

If you walk around a gym these days you will see many guys and gals working from a training programme. They may be following from an app on their phone or it may be written on a gym programme card.

This is great! By following a set routine, it will give the trainer a clear plan on what to do once they are in the gym. This is especially true for those who don't have a "study background" in anatomy and physiology, or are new to the whole training game.

However, from my experience I have noticed that in the majority of cases one of two things happens with trainers following a set routine:

First and the most common mistake is that after only a few weeks into this new training routine, the trainer will hear of another way to train that is "far better".

This will usually come about by seeing a cleverly marketed routine or stumbling across a thread on a forum written by someone whose avatar shows Mr Olympia striking a double bicep pose. Yeah! We have all been drawn in by this type of thing at some point or another.

A few examples that I could make up and probably start making a living from if I were unethical and any good at internet marketing would be things like: "Get abs in only 2 weeks!", "Build huge muscles with 3 minute workouts", "shocking breakthrough in muscle gain" or "Be Mr Olympia in less than a week!".

When we set out to achieve any goal, sure, we want the results "yesterday" and this is true for more than just results related to fitness. But the truth is:

"Anything that's worth having is never easy to get"

I personally, didn't start getting serious results from my weight training until I embraced the meaning of this quote to realise that there are no quick fixes, magic bullets or shortcuts that would lead me to the Holy Grail of "Quick muscle gain". But it's not just 100% hard work in the gym, you also have to train smarter..... But more on that later.

Needless to say, like most other people, I have been burned more than once in the past. But this was part of my learning curve, without learning from these mistakes; I would not be here right now.

The kinds of statements suggesting that there are short cuts to muscle gain, or that there are easy ways to get great results really do grate on me.

It is true that some trainers will have an easier ride with muscular development due to their genetic makeup but it takes time, consistency, correct diet and training for anyone (genetically gifted or otherwise) to achieve good results. And sadly many people are sold on the idea that they can get a quick fix when it comes to building muscle. If you are constantly looking to find "shortcuts" or "secrets" in your search for "instant muscle gain", you could be wasting years of real muscular development.

So, it's time to get your head in the right place, understand that there is no easy way and look to start working hard and smart in and out of the gym.

The second thing that can happen is that a trainer in search of fitness development will get a training programme that they like and follow it with no progression year in, year out. This does not yield great results either.

The trainer will reach a plateau and never progress. The result is often boredom and frustration causing them to take their foot off the gas and sometimes quit altogether. When training turns stagnant, and fitness results are non-existent, the repercussions from a mental and emotional point of view can be pretty devastating to a trainer that would otherwise have lots of potential.

But I guess you would like to know a bit more about me, who I am and why you should listen to me before you decide to take my advice? After all, I could be the guy on the forums with Arnolds bicep as my avatar!

I'm James Atkinson (Jim to my friends and readers) from jimshealthandmuscle.com. I started lifting weights when I was about fourteen and I am now into my thirties. I have been at both ends of the fitness scale, starting off as a small skinny kid.

I have been a long distance runner (Which does not help with muscle building), spent a number of years in an airborne unit in the British Army, a personal trainer and most recently, a competing bodybuilder.

I would like to pass on my experience to you and help you out with a full progressive year of weight training so you can get some real results! The training plan outlined in this book is the exact training plan that I designed and followed that gave me my first set of real bodybuilding results. And to this day, I still use the full routine and the principals in my own training.

Although this can be used for bodybuilders, it is a well-rounded routine that can be used for anyone. A few tweaks with diet and intensity, and it can be used for fat loss and general fitness alike.

I am not going to go on about how easy it is to pack on muscle and I am not going to tell you that I have the ultimate breakthrough answer to bodybuilding and fitness. Because I know for a fact that anyone claiming to have these "Magical formulas" are, let's say: "being economical with the truth".

Any successful, honest bodybuilder or weight trainer will tell you this. Maybe not in as many words but the meaning will be the same.

So:

- If you are looking to actually get some results and are willing to train hard and smart, this book is for you.
- If you have been lifting weights for a while and need a direction, you need not look elsewhere.
- If you are just starting out on your weight lifting or bodybuilding journey, I think you have done very well to find this. It will save you much time and frustration.

I will assume that you are not a complete beginner and that you have access to a good gym. If you do not have access to a gym and are a total beginner, you will still benefit from this course.

In fact, I have noticed that most mainstream gyms do not have trainers that actually train themselves to the level outlined in this book.

My advice here is to join a gym that has competing bodybuilders as members or staff. You will learn a huge amount about weightlifting and you will be exposed to the passion of these guys. This is only a good thing. A gym full of "meat heads" (no offence to fellow meat head intended) may be off putting to a lot of guys and gals that are new to the game but from my personal experience, nine out of ten "meat heads" will be friendlier than they look and are more than willing to help you out if you get stuck.

Helpful: If you are reading the digital version of this book you can take advantage of the links on the workout plans. Just click on the exercise that you are about to perform and you will be taken to the description page should you need a memory jogger of the correct technique. Remember that exercise form is king and you can't perfect this enough!

IMPORTANT, PLEASE READ:

Before we get started, I know that there is a full years training plan outlined in this book and this is probably the main reason that you made the purchase?

But please read the full book before you get started. I want you to actually get results, and there is a lot of information in the other content that will really help you along. This content can actually be the deciding factor in your training success.

The fundamentals are extremely important and if there are indeed any "magic formulas" for fitness or muscle building, this is where you will find them!

I would also like to point out that the training methods and concepts inside this book are the ideas that I have found to be most effective in my personal experience of nearly 20 years. Many other fitness professionals will however have their own ideas.

Health Check

Before you embark on any change of diet or fitness programme please consult your Doctor if you are unsure of the health implications these changes may have.

- If you are taking medication please check with you Doctor to make sure that it is ok for you to make these changes.

- If in any doubt at all please check with your Doctor first. It may be helpful to ask for a blood pressure, cholesterol and weight check. You can then have these read again in a few months after exercise or change of diet so you can monitor the benefit.

- It is also a good idea to take this workout routine with you and go through it with your doctor or physician. These guys will be able to tell you if there are any aspects that need changing based on your individual requirements.

Macro, meso, micro cycles

W hen working towards any muscle building goal, it is important to set out a good plan that stretches over a long period. It is also important that this plan is phased.

In this book we will split the year up into four phases. Each of these four phases are called meso cycles and the whole years training is known as a macro cycle. This whole planning process is known as "periodization" This in itself is a fundamental part of fitness that is hugely overlooked.

Now, this is just for your information and may be of interest but I do not want to overcomplicate this book by using too much jargon. My aim it to keep it simple and easy to follow.

An over view of the years training will be:

- A phase of "strength training"
- A phase of " 2 day split pre exhaust" training
- A phase of "2 day split compounds before isolations" training
- A phase of "3 day split" training

Don't worry if this doesn't make any sense yet, we will go over each phase in detail in the respective chapters.

Not Looking To Become A Bodybuilder?

If you are not looking to develop a huge bodybuilder physique, you will still benefit massively from this type of workout.

I truly believe that the mind-set and training methods of a successful bodybuilder is the key to any kind of fitness accomplishment. If you are looking to lose body fat or work on developing a tight physique in general, it is in this training environment that your focus should be.

Those guys and girls that you see on stage all tanned up looking vascular and insanely muscular didn't get that way by accident. That look is the result of extreme training and dieting. The same can also be said of the guys and girls that have visible muscle showing through their clothes that you see in everyday life when you are out and about.

As a personal trainer, when I had a potential new client, it would often be a "hard sell" for me to get them to start lifting weights as part of their training routine. The main reason for this was that the client believed that as soon as they started lifting weights, they would pack on a huge amount of muscle. This kind of mentality was very common, especially with the ladies.

I believe that the best mentality to have if you want to actually achieve fitness results in the form of muscular development is that of a bodybuilder. The term "muscular development" is fairly broad and by "muscular development, I mean any or all of the following:

- Muscle tone
- Muscle strength
- Muscle growth

So if you have picked up this book in the hope to tone up and lose body fat, but not necessarily build a huge hulk like physique, you are in the right place! For those reading this that do want to pack on slabs of muscle, you are also in the right place.

As you will find out later in the book (if you are not aware already), diet plays a huge part in your final result. It may sound like I am stating the obvious here but the food that you put into your body has a massive effect on your physique coupled with the training that you do.

If you are still sceptical about lifting heavy weights in the gym, I would like to point out a few other health benefits.

First off, I will be referring to the term "lean muscle" a bit throughout this book and I would like to clear up what I mean by this:

Lean muscle is bodyweight that is made up of functioning muscle. These muscles could be superficial and clear in plain sight or muscles that are deep and out of sight. So if you have plenty of lean muscle, it does not necessarily mean that you will have "huge muscles".

One of the most valuable properties of having a lot of lean muscle is that you will passively burn more calories. This means that you can burn more body fat by doing the same amount of exercise as someone that does not have lean muscle. In essence, you will be getting more value for your effort if you would like to reduce your levels of body fat.

The above argument in my "Hard sell" of using a weight training routine to potential "fat loss" clients was normally enough to convince them that lifting weights was a good idea.

But there are also many other benefits to lifting weights. One of the more major ones in my opinion is that a regular resistance routine will help to increase bone density. This will be an extra defence against fractures and along the same lines, weight training will also help to reduce the risk of osteoporosis which is common in many people during the ageing process.

These are great long term benefits which I feel are a very valuable investment in long term health.

The last thing that I would like to mention here is the work load of a weight training routine.

Another common scene in any gym, certainly the ones that I have been in, is what I like to call "Wasted workouts"

Fair play! The guys doing these "wasted workouts" have embraced the idea that they need to use weight training as part of their workout routine but they are not pushing themselves as much as they should be, by only going through the motions and lifting weights that are not challenging enough for them to actually get any development.

This is in my opinion a huge waste! The main problem here is that they have managed to motivate themselves enough to get up off the sofa and actually get to the gym to train, but this effort is cheated by not delivering a worthwhile outcome.

It's like having the opportunity to invest £1 to make £100 or having the opportunity to invest the same £1 to make £0.50p

Another great way to look at this is from a time perspective: It takes the same amount of time to do a "wasted workout set" as it does to do a worthwhile workout set, so you may as well make that set count.

For many people the hardest part of the whole fitness lifestyle is actually finding the time to get to the gym, so once you have jumped this hurdle, why not make the most of your time spent in the gym.

A lot of trainers that have not taken on a weight training routine before may find that lifting heavy weights is an idea that does not come naturally. I am fully aware of this but I would say that the longer you are in the muscle building game and the harder that you work; the more closer you will come to realising that building muscle is harder than you think.

So if you are looking to take on a weight lifting routine but don't want to be a huge bodybuilder. (Maybe you are just looking to burn some fat and tone up your body?) And happen to have found your way to this book, please don't be tempted to fall into the "wasted workout category" and use half of the weight that you are capable of lifting in your training sessions.

My experience has shown me that the bottom line is:

If you train like a bodybuilder, whatever your fitness goals might be, you will be happy with the result

Be Holistic And Structured

M aybe you have a burning desire to change your body shape completely and become as muscular as you can be? Or you may even want to take it to the next level and actually look into taking part in a bodybuilding competition at some point?

I know for many readers, some of the information here will not be new and these readers may have read similar things elsewhere. But I feel that there is not enough structure to weight lifting and bodybuilding routines available. I also believe that the correct planning and periodization of any weight lifting routine is a fundamental factor in the overall success.

As I mentioned in an earlier section, this planning is hugely overlooked. If you are a veteran weight lifter or bodybuilder and you do not plan your training phases to be progressive, this is something that will no doubt help you.

It's all well and good having a structured plan, but I also believe that you need to look at most weight lifting and bodybuilding routines in a holistic way.

For example, I have heard statements like the following too many times:

"I just need to lose this belly, so I need to work on my abs"

Or

"I just want to get bigger biceps, so I'm doing mostly bicep curls"

So the first guy who wants to lose a bit of belly fat does 500 crunches per day for six months and sees no change, he then believes that he will always have the belly fat; it's just the way he is

And the guy who wants bigger arms does bicep curls several times per week and sure, he gets some results, but now his body looks unbalanced

If these guys had been a bit smarter, looked at working their whole body and added the correct nutrition to their lifestyle; guy #1 would be leaner all over and because of these results, he would be motivated to continue with his fitness development. Guy #2 would have a balanced body and because he allowed more rest after each bicep training session, his biceps would be even bigger. As you can see, it is not just physical results that come from smart training.

It is with this holistic approach that you will get to know your own body. The longer that you embrace this idea, the better you will become. One of the great things about this is that you will get to know which of your muscle groups respond well and which of your muscle groups need a bit more attention.

It's a great feeling when you turn your weaknesses into your strengths!

Your Strength And Weakness As A Bodybuilder

When it comes to bodybuilding, many inspired trainers will have been subjected in some way to the all-time greats such as Reg Park, Arnold Schwarzenegger, Lee Haney, Ronnie Coleman, Jay Cutler and the list goes on.

These guys all have good genetics and have a head start when it comes to competition bodybuilding; they have good muscle structures and also height, giving them good proportions and symmetry. These guys will no doubt have their own weaknesses but they will have identified them early and moved mountains to bring them up to scratch.

It's not my intention to dishearten you, because it is certainly true that a guy holding down a full time job and family life can get amazing head turning results, but it is important to understand that the Mr Olympia title holders and such have been gifted with good genetics and to get this far, they have dedicated their whole lives to this sport often spending more money on food and supplements than the average household will even earn.

My point is that whoever you are, you can get great results, so don't let anything stop you from being the best that you can be!

I am one of the guys who some might call a "hardgainer". This means I was born with a small frame, average height and low body fat. A naturally skinny kid not designed for bodybuilding.

However, I don't like to use the term "hardgainer", so I call myself an "ectomorph" with average height. This didn't stop me from wanting to develop the best physique that I possibly could. And it should not stop you either if you are in the same boat as me.

You may however be someone who is gifted with good bodybuilding genetics. If this is the case, great stuff! But don't sit back and think that it will be easy. Being gifted with good genetics is one thing, but getting fitness results is another. You still need to put in the hard work.

I have seen many men and women that have got great genetics for competitive bodybuilding but sadly these guys don't have the slightest interest in the sport or even the gym, so they will never reach their potential.

It's all down to the individual to really want to change their body shape. A lot of bodybuilders that look amazing have put in a bunch of hard work to get their awesome physique but if they had better genetics their journey would have been different.

The bottom line is that yes, you may not be gifted in certain areas but by paying more attention and prioritizing these areas, you can build on your weakness. This is the great thing about the sport. One guy may have been at the front of the queue when the deltoid muscles were handed out but he may also have gotten to the chest muscle queue a bit too late. This guy will need to pay more attention and prioritize his chest muscles in his workouts.

If you feel that you have bad genetics when it comes to bodybuilding, you should not let this hold you back. If you are dedicated, train smart and hard, you will end up with better results and be looking better than the gifted guys that don't train as hard or smart.

Whether you are looking to compete in bodybuilding competitions or you would just like to develop an awesome physique, it is a good idea to identify any weak points that you may have early in the game.

If you are honest with yourself, it's pretty easy to look at yourself and pick out your weaknesses. For a bodybuilder, this is actually very important. If you can identify these weaknesses, you know what will let your physique down if you ever decided to compete.

I would go as far as to say that if you are going to commit to a bodybuilding lifestyle, the sooner that your weaknesses are identified, the better. You will then be able to start turning these weaknesses into strengths.

On the flip side of this coin, there are also guys that will have been working out for several years and have earned some results but will only be able to see their strong points.

A common example of this is: You may have had good gains in your biceps fairly quickly, as you have seen the gains here, you may dedicate more time to these to get them even bigger and end up neglecting your quads that are actually one of your natural weaknesses.

So your strong points get stronger and your weak points get weaker. The longer that you train like this the longer it will take to balance things out. And balancing everything out is one of the aims of this book

The above example is often what happens with many guys that start lifting weights. It is however in my personal experience the opposite way around with females. Women can often pick out their weaknesses right away.

If you happen to train in a gym that has experienced competition bodybuilders as members or employees and you would like to compete in the future or you just want a great balanced physique, it may be worth asking them to look at your frame and they may be able to point out where your natural weaknesses and strengths lie.

If you have not trained before and want to get into bodybuilding, it may be necessary to train each body part with the same intensity for six months to a year to help you identify weak areas or areas that are not responding as well as others.

Sometimes, it takes a period of consistent training to gain some visible results before you will recognise any muscle groups that might not respond as well to the training intensity that you are currently doing.

Most people will have certain muscle groups that will explode with growth and other muscle groups that will take a bit longer to develop. This is totally normal, but once you find these "lazy" muscle groups, you can look at different ways to "Motivate" them into development.

To Sum This Up

- Yes you may have weaknesses. Be honest with yourself and identify these.
- Maintain your strengths but build on your weaknesses.
- Don't be disheartened with the hand that you were dealt. You CAN get great results!
- If it is not yet clear where your strengths and weaknesses lie, give it a bit of time and try to focus on a balanced training routine until these emerge. (The yearlong routine in this book is a good place to start)

Plan Out Your Phases

———

Before you skip the next few sections of this book and flick to the training routines and rush off to get started, there are a few things that you need to do before you even think about going to the gym.

Mental attitude, preparation and planning are as important in this game as any set or rep that you will do in the gym!

I always find that the correct preparation for a new venture like this will help out massively and may also be a huge factor in actually seeing it through rather than getting side-tracked and starting another idea before any results are seen.

Remember that it takes time, consistency and effort to build a decent amount of muscle. I have seen so many people chop and change from one routine to the next within a matter of weeks and this seems to be common practice.

I think this stems from marketing strategies or "trends" on social media used to get a product into the hands of a buyer. This marketing strategy exploits the consumer by offering un realistic answers to their problem. In this case, quick results and minimal effort seem to be the common denominators here.

The best thing that you can do is to take what you have seen in muscle building magazines with a pinch of salt (If you actually step back and look at these magazines, you will notice that sometimes over 50% of the magazine is actually taken up by adverts for expensive supplements and equipment!

These kinds of media will often give you good advice or a solid 8-12 week routine but, the way these are written often make the reader feel that if they spend these few weeks following the programme, they will have undergone a great body transformation in this short time.

You are unlikely to read information that suggests it will take many months or even years of consistency before you get your results. The sooner that you start looking at bodybuilding as a long term process, the better.

I can guarantee that if you stick to the information in this book and see the full programme through, you will have a different body shape that you will be more than happy with a year from now.

Not only does planning a full years' worth of training give you a clear progressive direction, it will also make you feel motivated and ready to get started on your exciting muscle building journey.

You will have a countdown to the next phase, you can look forward to the upcoming change in training, and you will feel ready for the next phase when it hits. This is all to do with the mental preparation. It is easier to stick to a training programme if it is written down and there are dates involved.

So before we continue, grab your calendar or better still go to your digital calendar and block out each training phase.

Your macro cycle

FIRST OF ALL, YOU NEED to establish your start date and from this start date:

- Block out the next Twelve weeks with; "STRENGTH TRAINING".
- Block out the thirteenth week as "REST" (No training)
- Next, block out the fourteenth to twenty-fifth week as "2 DAY SPLIT PRE EXHAUST".
- Block out the twenty-sixth week as "REST" (no training)
- Block out week twenty-seven to week Thirty-eight as "2 DAY SPLIT COMPOUND BEFORE ISOLATION"
- Week Thirty-Nine is "REST"
- Block out weeks Forty to Fifty-one as "3 DAY SPLIT"
- Week Fifty-two is "REST"

You can then start this cycle again from the beginning the following year, but you will be bigger and stronger so you will have to adjust the weights that you use accordingly.

After each training phase there will be a week of rest so that your body has chance to recuperate and get ready for the next challenges.

Once these phases have been blocked out in your diary, you will have your start date. Next thing you will need to know is what to train, how to train and why you are training in this way for each phase.

This is exactly what we will cover in the next few sections.

Lifting with Correct Form

Using correct form when resistance training is in my opinion one of the major fundamentals in bodybuilding that is sacrificed all too often for heavier weight.

You may have heard the phrase "*Go heavy or go home*"? This is true to a certain extent, but you need to "*go as heavy as you can using the correct form.... Or go home*"

It doesn't have the same ring to it I know!

There is always someone in the gym (normally standing in the free weights area in front of the biggest mirror) with the 30kg dumbbells using their whole body to swing the heavy weights up to "Simulate" bicep curls.

This is terrible! Don't do this; it will not help you build muscle. If you want the maximum amount of value for your time spent in the gym, when you lift weights, you should hit the muscle that you are working with intensity. The more you can isolate the muscle group that you are working on, the better the results you will achieve.

If we take our friend who is trying to work his biceps by swinging the 30kg dumbbells for example; it is clear that he is not training his biceps efficiently. He is using momentum to complete the movement, yes he has a big weight but the movement is hugely diluted.

He would increase his gains exponentially if he were to drop the weight by 50% and work on his form so it was just his biceps doing the work. Sure this may damage his ego a bit but would he really need an ego if his biceps were nicely developed through correct lifting technique?

I'm not saying that you should go and start pumping iron with the 2kg. The key is to lift as heavy as you can but as soon as you notice that you are losing your form or that you feel that other muscles that you are not directly targeting are taking over, you should realise that this is your limit.

An example of this for me is on the bench press. I know when I have gone too heavy, because on each rep, I feel my shoulders taking most of the punishment.

Yeah, these muscles will be working harder, but I'm doing bench press to target my chest. If I want to target my shoulders I will do Shoulder press.

When this happens I just lower the weight and make sure I get a good set in that really hits my chest.

"It is more than ok to do one or two "Cheat reps" at the end of your set, but make sure that you are not doing "Cheat sets"!

You will occasionally get told that you are not lifting enough by your training partner or others in the gym but please understand that sacrificing good form for more weight is if anything diluting your overall results.

If you make it your priority to concentrate on good form and really get that pump in the muscle that you are working, in time you will agree with me 100%.

You should lift enough weight so that you are close to failure on the last 2 reps of your set whilst still maintaining good form.

It does help to have a training partner spotting you to help you through the last few reps.

The *"exercise descriptions"* section of this book has illustrated instructions of all of the movements that you will need to do this full year of bodybuilding. This will put you on the right track.

Take a look at this section and familiarise yourself on these exercises before attempting them.

It is always worth revisiting the descriptions from time to time as this will ensure that you do not fall in to bad habits.

Keep It Simple

———

During this year of training we will be keeping it simple and focusing on basic resistance movements. In my experience, this is the best way to get great results. I have seen many guys in the gym that have decided to follow an eight week routine that seems new and exciting, but I have also noticed that a lot of these routines are not actually designed to build muscle.

Many of these seemingly new ideas actually originate from other specialist fitness niches. They would work great if you were training to be a 100m sprinter, tennis player or something like that. But we are not training for track and field; we are training for resistance and bodybuilding. So there is very limited need for "Plyometric", "differential" and other track and field, and sport specific training methods.

We will stick to the "bread and butter" muscle building movements because these are all you will need to get your results.

Sure, these other methods can be added further down the line, but it is best to get the basics in place first.

If you have looked at the programme already, you may think it looks a bit daunting. But I can assure you that once you get used to this you will realise that this is all based around training the large muscle groups and although there are a fair few exercises, as you get into this, you will see that many of these exercises are similar movements but with slight variations.

Isolation and Compound movements explained

———

There are two types of resistance training that we are going to exploit in this year's programme. "Isolation movements" and "Compound movements"

Isolation

ISOLATION EXERCISES are movements that only involve one joint. A few examples of these are; Pec dec and pec flyes. These are for the chest muscles and things like lateral raises and front raises are examples of isolation exercises for the shoulders.

The body joint that is moving in both of these examples, is the shoulder joint. This type of exercise is arguably also known as a "shaping" exercise. Generally the weight that you are able to lift on isolation exercises will be considerably lighter than compound movements.

Compound

COMPOUND EXERCISES are big movements that use more than one joint in their execution.

Some classic examples of compound movements are squats, bench press, dead lift, shoulder press.

If we look at bench press for instance, we can see that there is more than one joint in operation. As you go through the movement, you will see that not only does your shoulder joint move but this exercise also brings in your elbows.

The weight that you can lift on compound exercises will usually be considerably more than on isolation exercises. Arguably, compound movements are known as "Building" exercises.

If you take a look at the "Correct form" section, you will see that I have marked the illustrated exercises as "Isolation" or "Compound. The more you train with weights, the more you will understand this concept.

Sort out your diet

———

There is no point in getting your training right, hitting your sessions with high intensity and getting insane pumps if you are not going to fuel your body correctly.

In this section we will look at a fairly simple formula that you can use as a starting point for building muscle.

Once you have your nutrients planned out, you can set out your daily meal plan. If you have an idea of how much of which type of food you should be eating and hit this each day along with your training, you can't really go wrong.

I will advise you on the formula that I have used on myself and my clients in the past that has given us great results.

I will spare you the details and just get down to the formula. I know most weight trainers and bodybuilders would rather train and eat than read!

This formula is widely used and it is just one way of working your diet out. Before you read any more, find out your weight in kilograms and your height in centimetres. Once you have done that, grab a notepad, pen and calculator.

It is well worth going through this as you read it. This may look complicated but it not as bad as you think.

Calculate your BMR

FIRST WE FIND OUT OUR "BMR" This stands for Basel metabolic rate. It is an estimate of the number of calories that we will burn if we stay at rest meaning no exercise at all:

(MALE) BMR =

(Height in CM X6.25) + (Wight in KG X9.99) – (Age X4.92) + 5

As females have a different make up, the calculation is slightly different, it looks like this:

(FEMALE) BMR

(Height in CM X6.25) + (Wight in KG X9.99) – (Age X4.92) – 161

Great! You should now have a figure. This represents the amount of calories that you are estimated to burn per day if you did nothing.

Harris-Benedict Equation

THIS REPRESENTS THE amount of calories that you are estimated to burn depending on your activity level As this book is about bodybuilding I will outline the figures that you will most lightly be using.

The three choices below are most relevant to this subject. If you plan to follow the training programme that I have suggested in the latter sections of this book, you should use the "Heavy exercise 6-7 days per week which is - **BMR X 1.725.**

Moderate exercise (3–5 days per week) Daily calories needed = BMR x 1.55

Heavy exercise (6–7 days per week) Daily calories needed = BMR x 1.725

Very heavy exercise (twice per day, extra heavy workouts) Daily calories needed = BMR x 1.9

So now you can work out this equation:

Take the figure that you got for your estimated BMR and times this by 1.725

This will give you the estimated amount of calories that you should be putting into your body every day.

Break Your Calories Down

NEXT, WE NEED TO SPLIT your total calorie intake down into carbohydrates, proteins and fats.

You should now have on your paper: Your BMR and a figure to represent your estimated total calories needed after using Harris-Benedict equation. It is this figure that we will use to give us a starting point.

We now need to break down this number into calories from protein, carbohydrates and fat

I have always worked with 65% carbohydrates, 25% protein and 10% fat for muscle building.

Below is an example of the calculation for someone needing 2500 calories, so whatever number your total calories happens to be, you can just swap the 2500 for your figure.

$$2500 \times 0.25 = 625 \text{ calories from Protein}$$

$$2500 \times 0.65 = 1625 \text{ calories from carbohydrates}$$

$$2500 \times 0.10 = 250 \text{ calories from fat}$$

So you should now know exactly how many calories you need to start with per day. This may seem like a lot at first, especially if you are not a big eater, but eating is a big part of building muscle.

You need to look on the packets of the food that you are eating to find out their nutrient contents, but it is worth taking the time to educate yourself on the nutrients of the food that will become a big part of your diet. This will make things easier in the long run.

When you plan your diet it may also be useful to know that

$$1 \text{ gram of protein} = 4 \text{ calories}$$

$$1 \text{ gram of carbohydrate} = 4 \text{ calories}$$

1 gram of fat = 9 calories

This should be all of the information that you need. It may look complicated and you may feel that you need a degree in mathematics to work this out. But if I can do it, anyone can. I actually failed the maths test several times in the fire-fighters entrance exam, thus I am now a bodybuilder and writer!

If you do struggle with the workings out of this for whatever reason, I will be more than happy to help you out, you can contact me on my blog or through the facebook page.

Supplements

————

When starting out on a "muscle building adventure", these days it is very easy to get caught up in the supplement market.

All you have to do is type into Google "How to build muscle" and you will be bombarded with an endless stream of adverts on products that will "help you get the muscle that you want".

Supplements do have a place in your bodybuilding journey but there are other things that you need to prioritize and get right before launching yourself into a health store and buying all of the protein, creatine, BCAA's etc which have the biggest, most ripped body on the labels.

First and foremost, supplements are "supplements". This means that they work as a small part of your diet. It is my opinion that protein shakes should be used in the following way:

Let's say that we have worked out the macronutrients that we need every day to build muscle and let's say for arguments sake that we need 294g of protein per day.

You could eat 294g of protein from tuna or chicken for example. This is not always convenient, so you could add in a measure of protein to substitute one of these meals. As you will probably be eating around six to seven times per day, one substitute protein and carb shake will not be too much of a problem. I would however advise that this is kept to no more than one substitute per day.

The other time that a protein and carb shake can be used as nutrients is directly after your training session. The advantage of this is that the nutrients in many high quality protein shakes will be absorbed into your system quicker as it is part digested and therefore fast acting. This way, you are feeding your muscles the nutrients that they are crying out for directly after your workout.

Which protein shake to choose?

AS MENTIONED BEFORE there are thousands of brands of protein drinks that all claim that they are your best choice. It's probably true that many of the companies selling these will offer you a quality product, but it is also true that as many will probably offer you a choice that is of low quality and a waste of money.

The best thing to do is to look at the ingredients of these products before you buy them. The main thing that you are looking for is the content of "Whey protein" that is in your potential product.

Whey protein is a great source of quality protein that can be used for us bodybuilders. This is the source of the Branch chain amino acids that you see advertised on many supplements. Whey protein also contains small proteins known as peptides that increase blood flow to the muscles. It is for this reason that a Whey protein supplements should be consumed right after your training sessions.

Many of the protein shakes on the market today will also have things like creatine added. This may be a selling point but in my opinion it is more important that you are getting a quality whey protein supplement.

If you are to use these types of supplements, you should look at your dietary needs. You will have probably seen "Diet Protein drinks". In my experience, all this means is that this type of supplement is made up of less carbohydrates.

When choosing a protein powder it is worth looking not only at the whey protein content but at the amount of carbohydrates too as these will have an effect on your total calorie intake.

To sum this up

WHEN CHOOSING A PROTEIN shake:

- Make sure that you get a quality one. Don't be fooled by clever marketing. There are many supplements across a large price range that will do exactly the same job.

- Check the level and quality of Whey protein in the product

- Check the carbohydrate content. A product that says "Diet" will often mean it is low in carbohydrates

- Remember that protein shakes have an amount of calories in them and if you are sticking to a diet, you will want to add the calories that come from these shakes in

- Remember that an expensive product does not always mean good quality

The Use Of Creatine

———

Y ou will no doubt have heard of creatine being used for building muscle. I have personally had some good results from this supplement and thought I would share my experience as it fits in very well with this book.

Creatine is a great supplement. I have used this in many different ways. But the best way to use creatine that I have found for building muscle is outlined in this section.

There are several different types of creatine but I want to talk about "creatine Monohydrate".

Creatine monohydrate is normally the cheapest on the market and it has been very effective for me.

To Load Or Not To Load?

THERE ARE MIXED VIEWS when it comes to supplementing with creatine monohydrate. The biggest argument is whether or not to do a "Loading phase" with this product. To clarify, a loading phase is taking the creatine in a higher dosage during the first week or 5-7 days of the cycle. Some people suggest that this has no benefit. I have heard of people having stomach upsets from doing this also.

As I am in to finding the best results for me, I have tried both methods and also other suggested methods. But the best results have come from using a loading phase.

My greatest results came from the following plan....

Creatine Monohydrate Plan

———

- Week 1:

LOADING PHASE - 5g taken 5 times every day for 7 days

- Week 2 through to and including week 6:

MAINTENANCE PHASE - 5g taken 2 times every day for 7 days

- Week 7:

TAPERING PHASE - 5g taken 2 times 4 days of this week (Every other day)

- Week 8

TAPERING PHASE - 5g taken 2 times 3 days of this week (I did Mon, Wed, Fri)

When I use creatine monohydrate now, this is always the plan I follow. It gives me great results. I feel good effects (Fuller and stronger) by about week 3.

You will notice that there is a "Tapering phase" on this plan. I use this because I have in the past had great results but stopped and very quickly lost my gains and the effect of the creatine. By putting this tapering phase in, I noticed that I did not lose the gains I had achieved. After the 8 weeks I will have 6 weeks off and then "Rinse and repeat".

Another argument is that you do not have to cycle creatine. I can see why you would want to use it the full year through but personally I think it is good to give your body a rest from this supplement. If not for health reasons, for the health of your wallet!

To Sum Creatine Monohydrate Up

CREATINE MONOHYDRATE is a supplement that I really rate. I have had some good results with this. It is one of the cheapest types of creatine on the market. It is a good idea when buying a creatine monohydrate product to get it from a reputable source. As you may know there are a massive amount of companies and brands that get away with selling low quality products at high prices. A good indicator when looking for a creatine monohydrate product is if you can see the word "Creapure" on the label. I wouldn't waste money on something that wasn't a creapure brand. I have used this product with good effect; it's a good choice, cheap but good quality

I will also point out that this plan is the best that I have found works for me. There has been a lot of trial and error but if you are thinking of using creatine, you could use it as a starting point.

Optimise each training session

———

If you have been lifting weights for a while and you have "googled" things like:

"How to build muscle" or "best way to build muscle fast" you will have probably found articles relating to food intake, rest, and intensity of training. The advice in this section is probably advice that you have heard before, but it may be worth a read as it is always important to revisit the basics.

Building muscle is complicated, hard work and requires a lot of discipline. There are a lot of factors that you have to consider. If you have a solid training programme and a good bodybuilding diet, you are off to a good start!

You will also need to look at a few other things to get better results.

Sleep and rest

MUSCLE IS BUILT WHEN you rest. When you sleep, your body recovers through protein synthesis. This is basically, your body using the protein that you have given it to build muscle. It is good to eat something like cottage cheese or a slow release protein shake before you go to bed to further exploit this.

During sleep, your body also releases growth hormone so it is important that you get a good night sleep whenever you can. You should look to get a solid 8 hours.

Don't drag your workout out

WHEN TRAINING, YOU should try to limit your time in the gym. By this I mean that you should stick to your routine but you should keep it short and sharp.

If you have a lot to do in your routine, you should reduce time between sets and exercises. If you are trying to build muscle, there is really no need to train for longer than 1 hour per session. 1 hour 30 at max.

Remember that burning more calories, means having to put more calories back into your body for your muscles to grow. So train with intensity. If you have more exercises to do, you have less time to rest between sets.

Stay hydrated

IF YOU ARE FULLY HYDRATED when it comes to "workout o'clock" you will have a good workout. Proper hydration is vital if you want to get the most out of your training sessions. Being hydrated will allow you to perform a whole lot better on every rep of every set.

I personally drink a lot of water throughout the day and I really do notice it if I slack off on the water when it comes to my training session. To stay hydrated, you need to drink plenty of water all day, every day, not just ten minutes or so before a workout.

There are some good supplemental hydration drinks on the market but these can be expensive and you should not use them as your main source of hydration. Plain old water is where it's at! But feel free to add a slice of lemon or some other citrus fruit to your water for a bit of flavour if you wish.

Stay focused

THE GYM CAN BE A VERY social place. This is great, but you should not let the social aspect take from the main reason that you are there. The longer that you stand around chatting, texting, taking selfies, the longer your workout routine will take. This can be very detrimental to your development.

If you are following the routine outlined in this book, focus will be paramount, especially after the first phase. You will have a lot to get through and a lack of focus could make the workout drag on way longer than it should. This can cause loss of muscular gains. So when you are in the gym, be there to train.

I find that on my journey to the gym, if I visualise the exercises and the order I will be doing them in, it really puts me in the right frame and this mental preparation is where the focus starts for me.

Add some cardio

MANY WEIGHT LIFTERS/ bodybuilders see cardio as a "Gains killer" and the evil twin of muscle building. But I tend to disagree. Sure, if you are looking to build muscle and you are also training for long distance or marathon running, you will have a hard time gaining that muscle. But several cardio training sessions per week can only help. These sessions could be steady state or interval training.

If you take regular cardio exercise (three to four sessions per week) your body will become more efficient at functioning. This means that it will process nutrients better, recover better and also, when it comes to reducing body fat, you will see results a lot faster.

I would suggest that you try doing three to four 20-30 minute interval or steady state sessions per week. If you are interested in running training, you will find some good ideas including interval training advice in my book: *"Marathon training and distance running tips"*[1]

The truth is; the idea that cardio kills gains has been taken too literally by most bodybuilders/weight lifters. Remember that it is harder than you think to burn your hard earned muscle away with cardio sessions, and the pros of regular cardio training when it comes to building muscle far outweigh the cons.

Use a pre workout meal/ supplement

YOU SHOULD DEFINITELY plan to eat before each workout. By getting on top of this, you will have better training sessions, not just from a functional perspective but from a psychological point of view too.

There are thousands of pre workout drinks and supplements out there for you to spend your cash on, but I feel that the best pre workout nutrients that you can have comes from real food.

---

1. *http://www.amazon.com/Marathon-Training-Distance-Running-Tips-ebook/dp/B00LSPCVM6/*

ref=sr_1_3?ie=UTF8&qid=1428464704&sr=8-3&keywords=james+atkinson

Instead of spending an obscene amount of money on pre workout supplements, you should take advantage of the real food that will fuel your workout a whole lot better.

Any one or a combination of the following are perfect for fuelling your workouts:

- Fruit Smoothies
- Bananas
- Oats
- Wholegrain bread

This is by no means an exhausted list. These are just a few good choices based on their nutritional properties. When selecting a pre workout meal, you should look for a combination of foods that have slow release energy like oats. This type of food will keep you energised for longer. You should also look for something to give you a quick burst, like bananas and other fast acting carbohydrates. To round this off, you may want to look at getting some protein in to the mix to help repair as soon as you run your body down.

If you are not that clued up on nutrition and food groups, it is a great idea to invest a bit of time into learning. Education and self-education, if gleaned from a reliable source is the way to go here. The time you spend on this type of self-improvement is time well spent.

Here is an example of one of my pre workout meals:

- 1 cup of oats
- 1 scoop of whey protein
- 1 banana

This is a nice balance; these foods are also easy to throw in a blender to make a quick shake.

Some energy drinks and pre workout drinks have their place but I feel that they should not be the #1 priority when it comes to pre workout nutrition.

A lot of trainers will be drawn to pre workout supplements because of the intense buzzing and tingling feeling that these give, making them feel "wired" and focused. But here is a little secret:

This feeling most likely comes from two ingredients that are in the supplement. The first ingredient being caffeine and the other one being vitamin B3 (otherwise known as "niacin").

Both of the above ingredients can be bought fairly cheaply from any health store in pill form. But if you do decide to go down this road, please do not substitute a few pills for good honest food. Also please check with a physician or doctor to make sure these things are not detrimental to your health.

Use a post workout meal/ supplement

IF YOU HAVE DONE ANY kind of research on bodybuilding and weight lifting, you will know that your post workout meal is one of the most important meals that you need.

This is because after your workout, your body has been shocked. The workouts in this book or any type of demanding workout for that matter will put a lot of stress on the trainer's nervous system and if the trainer does not give their body what it needs, their body will suffer.

If this vital nutritional window is missed, the trainer could actually be breaking down muscle rather than building it. That seems like a massive waste of a training session to me!

As soon as you finish a workout, you should get this meal in. It is important to act quickly as your metabolism will be on fire and ready to process the nutrition that it needs.

You need fast absorbing carbohydrates and protein. The best carbohydrates are the more simple ones. I don't mean a few spoonful's of sugar. There is a nutrient called "dextrose" this is where post work out carbs are at!

You also need fast acting protein. The best form of fast acting protein is "Whey" protein. This is very widely available in powder form.

Luckily for us, there are plenty of post workout drinks available that take care of this specific combination of carbs and protein. So you may have guessed that the next thing that I will advise is that you get yourself a post workout protein and carbs drink to take as soon as you finish your training session.

When selecting a post workout shake, make sure that it is a high quality whey protein and it has dextrose as an ingredient.

There are a lot of different types of protein shakes available and some are more ideal for convenient meal replacements. The carbs in a lot of these are actually finely ground oats and as oats are slow release carbs, these are not ideal for post workout meals.

To sum this up; Post workout meals are extremely important. You should look at investing in a high quality post workout shake made up of dextrose and whey protein. Do not get confused with the different types of protein shakes/ meal replacements out there.

A Final Note Before You Get Started

―――――

I have designed this year's routine around a theory that I have put into practice myself and out of all of the training methods that I have tried, this has been the most successful for me.

Before each of the 12 week routines, I will explain why that part is set out the way it is. I think that it is important that you know why you are training in a certain way as you will know what to expect as an outcome.

Stick to the plan

EVERYONE MISSES THE odd training session. This will not "break the bank" at this stage. If you do get sick or miss a week or so of training, this is not the end of the world, but It is important that you stick to the plan and your dates for training progression changes.

Let's say that in the first 12 weeks you are unable to train for whatever reason at, let's say week five. Don't say to yourself;

"That's a week that I have missed, I will run this stage of training over an extra week"

There are two reasons for this;

The first is that, if you are on a tight schedule, you will be more likely to stick to your sessions. If I am involved in a training programme, I know that if I didn't train as hard as I should have before the next progression hits, I will struggle and will not be adequately prepared to take the next step.

The second reason is that if you do miss a week here and there and decide to add this onto the end, and run this training phase into the next training phase, there is a danger that you will never actually get onto the next progression. I have seen this done many times before.

If you never make it to your next progression, your results will not progress. If you only put in 50% of the training sessions, you will only get 50% of the results.

This is why you need to write it down and stick to your plan.

First 12 Weeks (Strength Training Phase)

———

You may think that this phase is not appropriate for you. If so, I would urge you not to skip this part. It is very important to do this phase as it will build you a strong foundation.

This first 12 weeks, we are going to concentrate on big compound movements. This is to build strength in all of the big muscle groups.

Remember to keep your form and lift as heavy as you can whilst sticking to the set and rep range.

Ideally, you want to be hitting failure on the 10th rep of the 3rd set. When this happens, you have found the weight that you need to work with.

If you have a training partner, you can hit failure on your 8th rep and allow them to help you with the last 2 reps.

The order that the exercises are listed in, is the ideal order in which to train, however at this point it will not cause too many problems with small deviations to this:

The first 12 week period looks like this:

WARM UP - 10 MINUTES on the cross trainer

Sets and reps: 3 sets of 10 reps

Training days: Monday, Wednesday, Friday

- **Flat bench press**
- **Lat Pull downs**
- **Bent over rows**
- **Leg press**
- **Bicep curls**
- **Shoulder press**
- **Tricep dips**
- **Crunches - _(optional)_**

Please check the exercise descriptions section if you are not sure of an exercise. It is also worth using this as a reference guide. Check back regularly to make sure that you are still lifting with correct form.

It really helps to plan you sessions and actually have a physical copy of your training plan pinned up somewhere that you will see it a lot in your everyday life. This little trick should not be underestimated. I have taken the liberty of creating a training chart that can be marked after every session.

The following chart can be copied, cut out (if you have the paperback version of the book) or you can create your own. Feel free to contact me for a PDF version, I will gladly sort you one out.

You will notice that on the chart, I have already marked your future gym visits for this training phase with a tick. Once you have completed a training session, you can mark the chart where the tick that represents the training session that you have just done is. Use a strikethrough, or even black out the full block.

This is a great tool for accountability and self-motivation. Here is the chart:

Strength Training
(Phase 1)

Monday	Tuesday	Wednesday	Thursday	Friday
✓		✓		✓
✓		✓		✓
✓		✓		✓
✓		✓		✓
✓		✓		✓
✓		✓		✓
✓		✓		✓
✓		✓		✓
✓		✓		✓
✓		✓		✓
✓		✓		✓

Second 12 Weeks 2 day Split (Pre exhaust Phase)

After the first 12 weeks of strength training, we should respond to this next phase very well. We will have built a fair bit of strength up and are now ready to start using that strength to chisel some muscle and target a bit more precisely.

We are going to be using isolation exercises before we do our compound movements. This is known as "Pre-exhaust" sets.

The theory behind pre exhaust sets is simple. If you isolate the muscle and wear it out, when you come to do your big compound movement on that muscle, it will have to work harder to lift the weight. If this kind of training is done for a fair length of time, (let's say 12 weeks!) your body will adapt and will become even stronger and developed than before.

Important

YOU WILL PROBABLY NEED to re assess the weight that you lift on your compound exercises when you first start training in this way.

The transition from the first stage to this one can really mess with your head at first. You will notice that the amount of weight that you were lifting on your compound movements in the previous weeks may have dropped quiet significantly.

This is normal. It is easy to think that you are taking backward steps but you need to realise that your body is not used to training in this way.

You are pre exhausting your muscle group before you hit your presses, this means that your muscles are really struggling through the exercises. And what's more you are making them do extra reps.

Please don't be tempted to sacrifice form for weight at this point. Push yourself yes, but always remember that if you dilute the movement by using incorrect form you are diluting your results.

The first few weeks of this stage will probably be the toughest as it will take time for your body to adapt. But towards the end of this 12 week cycle, you will be even stronger and bigger than before. You will be very surprised at what you can lift on a bench press when starting from fresh after this stage.

Important

IT IS NOW IMPORTANT that you stick to the exercise order in which they are listed. You need to make sure that you are doing an isolation exercise for a muscle group directly followed by a compound movement to ensure that you are challenging your muscles in the correct way.

The second 12 week period looks like this:

4 TRAINING SESSIONS per week preferably 2 days on 1 off, 2 days on and 2 off

An ideal example would be:

Workout A on Mondays & Thursdays

Workout B on Tuesdays & Fridays

Rest days Wednesdays, Saturdays & Sundays

4 sets of 12 to 8 reps

Workout A

- **Warm up - 10 minutes on the cross trainer**
- **Pec fly**
- **Bench press**
- **Lat pull-down**
- **Bent over rows shoulder with grip**
- **Close grip rows**
- **Tricep push down on Cables**
- **Tricep dips (Reasonable failure)**
- **Crunches (Reasonable failure)**

Workout B

- **Warm up - 10 minutes on the cross trainer**
- **Bicep curl**
- **Lateral raises with dumbbells**
- **Shoulder press**
- **Leg extensions**
- **Leg press**
- **Lying leg curl**

- **Calf raises**

PLEASE CHECK THE EXERCISE descriptions section if you are not sure of an exercise. It is also worth using this as a reference guide. Check back regularly to make sure that you are still lifting with correct form.

As this is a new phase, you will need a new "Accountability and motivation chart". As per the previous strength training phase, I have taken the liberty of creating a chart for you to use to keep track of your training.

As this is a 2 day split routine, I have set it up so that the training days are Monday, Tuesday and Thursday and Friday and used "Workout – A" or "Workout – B" instead of ticks. After each training session, strikethrough or block out on the chart the session that it represents.

Feel free to make your own version of this chart if your training days have to be different.

Here is the chart for your first 2 day split phase (Pre exhaust):

Pre- Exhaust Training
(Phase 2)

Monday	Tuesday	Wednesday	Thursday	Friday
Workout - A	Workout - B	REST	Workout - A	Workout - B
Workout - A	Workout - B	REST	Workout - A	Workout - B
Workout - A	Workout - B	REST	Workout - A	Workout - B
Workout - A	Workout - B	REST	Workout - A	Workout - B
Workout - A	Workout - B	REST	Workout - A	Workout - B
Workout - A	Workout - B	REST	Workout - A	Workout - B
Workout - A	Workout - B	REST	Workout - A	Workout - B
Workout - A	Workout - B	REST	Workout - A	Workout - B
Workout - A	Workout - B	REST	Workout - A	Workout - B
Workout - A	Workout - B	REST	Workout - A	Workout - B
Workout - A	Workout - B	REST	Workout - A	Workout - B

Third 12 Weeks, 2 Day SPLIT (Compound Before Isolation Phase)

———

This phase is where you see that you have actually become stronger as we will be doing our compounds first.

You will find that you can now bench press, shoulder press etc more than you could when you started. The first time that I did this routine, I found that my dumbbell shoulder press had gone up from 30kg to 40kg! I could actually shoulder press the 40kg dumbbells using very good form.

Remember that the weight on your isolation exercises may reduce slightly. If it does, do not be tempted to sacrifice your good lifting technique.

Your muscles will again respond well to the increase of weight from your compound exercises and the change from the pre exhaust style of training in the previous 12 week period.

Important

IT IS NOW IMPORTANT that you stick to the exercise order in which they are listed. You need to make sure that you are doing a compound exercise for a muscle group directly followed by an isolation movement to ensure that you are challenging your muscles in the correct way.

The third 12 week period looks like this:

4 TRAINING SESSIONS per week preferably 2 days on 1 off, 2 days on and 2 off

An ideal example would be:

Workout A on Mondays & Thursdays

Workout B on Tuesdays & Fridays

Rest days Wednesdays, Saturdays & Sundays

4 sets of 12 to 8 reps

Workout A

- **Warm up - 10 minutes on the cross trainer**
- **Bench press**
- **Cable crossovers**
- **Bent over barbell rows (Shoulder width grip)**
- **Close grip rows**
- **Lat pull-down**
- **Tricep dips**
- **Tricep pushdowns (cables)**
- **Swiss ball crunches**

Workout B

- **Warm up - 10 minutes on the cross trainer**
- **Bicep curls**
- **Shoulder press**
- **Lateral raises with Dumbbells**
- **Shrugs**
- **Leg press**
- **Leg extensions**

- Lying leg curl
- Calf raises

PLEASE CHECK THE EXERCISE descriptions section if you are not sure of an exercise. It is also worth using this as a reference guide. Check back regularly to make sure that you are still lifting with correct form.

Here is a new accountability chart for this phase. As the training sessions do not change, The same chart layout as the previous can be used here. But it is still a good idea to have a new chart as it signifies a new phase.

Here is your accountability and motivation chart for your third phase:

Compound Before Isolation Training (Phase 3)

Monday	Tuesday	Wednesday	Thursday	Friday
Workout - A	Workout - B	REST	Workout - A	Workout - B
Workout - A	Workout - B	REST	Workout - A	Workout - B
Workout - A	Workout - B	REST	Workout - A	Workout - B
Workout - A	Workout - B	REST	Workout - A	Workout - B
Workout - A	Workout - B	REST	Workout - A	Workout - B
Workout - A	Workout - B	REST	Workout - A	Workout - B
Workout - A	Workout - B	REST	Workout - A	Workout - B
Workout - A	Workout - B	REST	Workout - A	Workout - B
Workout - A	Workout - B	REST	Workout - A	Workout - B
Workout - A	Workout - B	REST	Workout - A	Workout - B
Workout - A	Workout - B	REST	Workout - A	Workout - B

Forth 12 Week 3 Day Split

———

The fourth and final 12 week period is a 3 day split. This means we lose a rest day and therefore are training 6 days of the week.

You will also notice that we are going back to isolation before compound exercises. It is important that you understand that you may have to drop your working weight on your compound exercises again.

Remember that you are still stressing your muscles enough for them to grow if you are reaching failure with a lighter weight on the same rep as you were when lifting a heavier weight in the previous 12 week period.

You are "Pre-exhausting" your muscles, so they have already had a good workout before you start doing your presses.

Before you get used to this idea, you may think that you are taking a backward step. Always keep in mind that you are not training to be a power lifter.

The fourth 12 week period looks like this:

6 TRAINING SESSIONS per week preferably 3 days on 1 off, 3 days on

4 sets of 12 to 8 reps:

Workout A

- **Warm up - 10 minutes on the cross trainer**
- **Cable crossovers**
- **Flat barbell press**
- **Incline barbell press**
- **Concentration curls**
- **Barbell curls**
- **Lying leg curls**
- **Stiff legged deadlifts**
- **Swiss ball crunches**

Workout B

- **Warm up - 10 minutes on the cross trainer**
- **Lateral cable raises**
- **Bent over dumbbell raises**
- **Barbell shoulder press**
- **Leg extensions**
- **Leg press**
- **Barbell squats**
- **Standing calf raises**

Workout C

- **Warm up - 10 minutes on the cross trainer**
- **Lat pulldowns**
- **Close grip row**
- **Bent over barbell rows (Hands shoulder width apart)**
- **Shrugs**
- **Tricep pushdowns**
- **Tricep dips**
- **Swiss ball crunches**

PLEASE CHECK THE EXERCISE descriptions section if you are not sure of an exercise. It is also worth using this as a reference guide. Check back regularly to make sure that you are still lifting with correct form.

Your last chart is set up in the same format as the other 2 day split routines but this time using 6 training days and one rest day on a seven day chart. Check it off as you go

Here is your last accountability and motivational chart for your 3 day split:

3 Day Split
(Phase 4)

Monday	Tuesday	Wednesday	Thursday	Friday	Saturday	Sunday
Workout - A	Workout - B	Workout - C	REST	Workout - A	Workout - B	Workout - C
Workout - A	Workout - B	Workout - C	REST	Workout - A	Workout - B	Workout - C
Workout - A	Workout - B	Workout - C	REST	Workout - A	Workout - B	Workout - C
Workout - A	Workout - B	Workout - C	REST	Workout - A	Workout - B	Workout - C
Workout - A	Workout - B	Workout - C	REST	Workout - A	Workout - B	Workout - C
Workout - A	Workout - B	Workout - C	REST	Workout - A	Workout - B	Workout - C
Workout - A	Workout - B	Workout - C	REST	Workout - A	Workout - B	Workout - C
Workout - A	Workout - B	Workout - C	REST	Workout - A	Workout - B	Workout - C
Workout - A	Workout - B	Workout - C	REST	Workout - A	Workout - B	Workout - C
Workout - A	Workout - B	Workout - C	REST	Workout - A	Workout - B	Workout - C
Workout - A	Workout - B	Workout - C	REST	Workout - A	Workout - B	Workout - C
Workout - A	Workout - B	Workout - C	REST	Workout - A	Workout - B	Workout - C

Rinse and repeat

———

Once that you have completed your years training routine, you can progress in many ways from here.

You could rinse and repeat, by this I mean start again from the beginning. It is more than ok to do this as you will be further challenging your muscles.

You will more than likely find that you can lift a lot more on the first 12 weeks this time around than you could when you first started.

By this point you may even have identified your weak points or certain muscle groups that are not developing as quickly as others. If you are in this position, you can still use this routine as a guide. I suggest that you prioritize your weak areas or add an exercise or two for that muscle group.

By prioritize, I mean train these weaker muscle groups at the beginning of your workouts when you are fresh.

The longer you are in the game for, the better development you will receive. Not only will this be muscular development, but you will also learn more about your own body's reaction to certain types of training.

The outcome to this will be an efficient training routine that is personal to you. You will only get to this point by starting out with a solid general plan, seeing it through and reassessing at the end, hence the whole idea of this book.

There are many ways to upgrade your training routine. Some of these include:

- Increasing weight
- Changing rep range
- Reducing time between sets
- Changing exercises
- Changing exercise order
- Adding exercises for weaker muscle groups

- Reducing exercises for stronger muscle groups to allow for increased work on weaknesses
- Focus on a single muscle group per training session.

Exercise descriptions

In this section I have included illustrated descriptions of the exercise and how to perform it correctly.

I would advise that you use this as your "go to "guide. It will do you no harm to revisit this section from time to time to ensure that you are getting the best out of your training.

Flat bench press

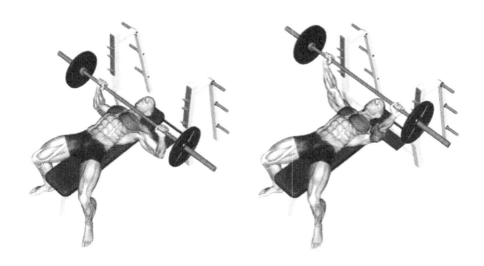

COMPOUND EXERCISE TARGETING Chest muscles

Start Position: Lay on a flat bench under a barbell on a rack or smiths machine so that your eyes are in line with the bar. Form a right angle with your arms. This will form your grip width, now grip the bar.

Movement: Lift the bar off the rack or unhook from a smiths machine and straighten your arms. As you inhale, lower the bar down to meet your mid chest. As the bar touches your mid chest, exhale and push the bar back up to the start position.

You should complete this with a "2 second up, 2 second down tempo". This will ensure that you are getting the most out of the exercise.

Lat Pull downs

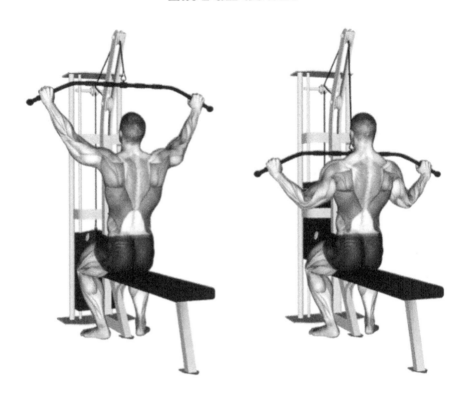

Compound exercise targeting: Back muscles (Lats)

START POSITION: Make sure that any thigh pads are adjusted to rest comfortably across your thighs and your feet are flat on the floor. Stand up and grip the bar so your hands are in line with the outside of your shoulders, then take at least one hand space further out. (I use 2 hand spaces. If this movement feels tight on your shoulders, try taking another hand space out).

Movement: Keeping this grip, step back into the machine and sit down. Look at the top of the machine throughout the exercise. As you exhale, pull the bar down, below your chin to meet your upper chest. Inhale as you return to the start position.

You should complete this with a "2 second up, 2 second down tempo". This will ensure that you are getting the most out of the exercise.

Bent over rows (Shoulder width grip)

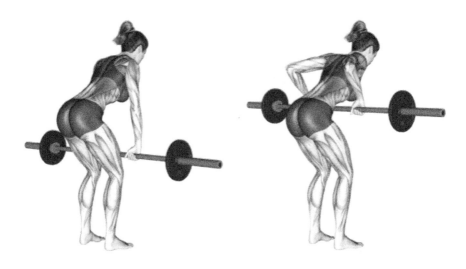

Compound exercise targeting: Back muscles (Lats)

START POSITION: Place your bar on the floor and stand in front of it with your feet shoulder width apart and toes turned out slightly. Keeping your knees bent and back flat, bend over and pick up the bar. Grip the bar so your hands are in line with your outer shoulders and take a further hand space wider but no more than this.

Keeping your knees bent and back flat, stand up straight with the bar. If you need to at this point, you can adjust the width of your feet so that it is comfortable. Keeping your back flat and knees bent, lower the bar so that it hangs below your knees.

Movement: As you exhale, bring the bar up so that it touches your belly button, your elbows should go higher than your back and it is important that your back is kept flat. (I find that when doing rows, if I concentrate on pushing my chest forward at the top of the movement it helps to keep my back flat). As you inhale, lower the bar back to the starting position

You should complete this with a "2 second up, 2 second down tempo". This will ensure that you are getting the most out of the exercise.

Leg press

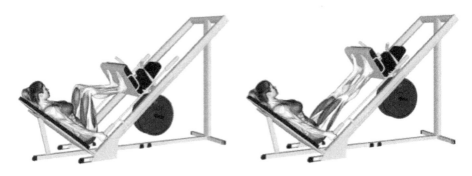

Compound exercise targeting: Leg muscles (Quads)

START POSITION: Adjust your seat of the machine that you are using if it has this option. Sit on the machine and place your feet on the upper section of the foot plate. Your feet should be about hip width apart and toes slightly turned out. It is important that your feet stay flat on the foot plate throughout the movement. (If you struggle to keep your heels flat, you may want to move your feet further up the foot plate.)

Movement: when you are good to go, take the weight and unhook the carriage. As you exhale, straighten your legs to the point just before they lock. DO NOT LOCK YOUR LEGS OUT. Inhale and lower the weight down so your legs form a right angle. As you exhale, return to the start position.

(Some people may be able to go lower than a right angle, by doing this you will also be working the glute muscles more. If you do try this just be aware of the strain that you are putting on your hips and knees, if you do start to feel pain in these areas, return to right angles)

You should complete this with a "2 second up, 2 second down tempo". This will ensure that you are getting the most out of the exercise.

Bicep curls

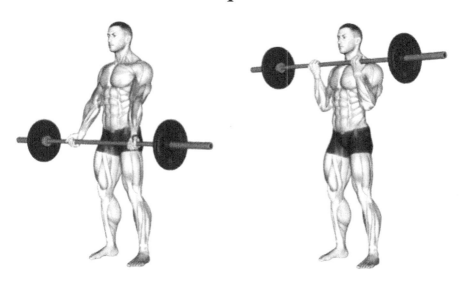

Isolation exercise targeting: Front upper arm muscles

START POSITION: When picking up your bar, ensure that your knees are bent and back is flat. When gripping the bar, your palms should be facing up and your hands should be shoulder width apart. Stand up straight, elbows slightly bent NOT LOCKED OUT and you are ready to begin.

Movement: As you exhale, bring your forearms up until they are at a right angle to the floor, at this point, in one movement, push your elbows forward to bring your hands closer to the front of your shoulders. At maximum contraction, inhale as you lower the bar back to the start position.

You should complete this with a "2 second up, 2 second down tempo". This will ensure that you are getting the most out of the exercise.

Shoulder press

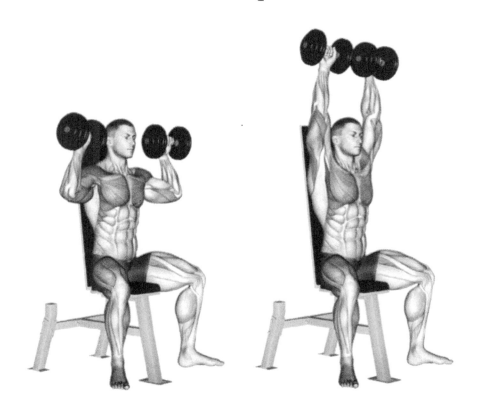

Compound exercise targeting: Shoulder muscles

START POSITION: It is best to do these facing a mirror. You should use an adjustable bench and set this so it is just under maximum upright position (1 notch back). Grab your dumbbells and sit on the bench resting them on their ends on your quads. Bring the dumbbells up to chin level and turn your palms so they are facing forward. (You may need a training partner to help with this)

Movement: As you exhale, push the dumbbells up above your head so they meet just before your elbows lock out. DO NOT ALLOW YOUR ELBOWS TO LOCK OUT AT THE TOP OF THE MOVEMENT. Inhale as you return to the start position.

You should complete this with a "2 second up, 2 second down tempo". This will ensure that you are getting the most out of the exercise.

Tricep dips

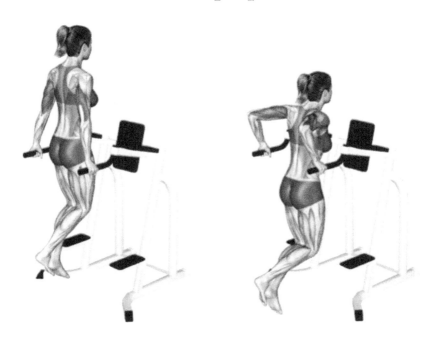

COMPOUND EXERCISE TARGETING: Rear upper arms (Triceps)

Start position: Take a grip of your dips bars so your hands are in line with your shoulders. Take the weight of your body onto your arms. Ensure that your arms are not locked out straight, you should have them slightly bent. Your legs should hang down below you or you can bend your knees, bringing your heals up towards your glutes.

Movement: As you inhale, lower your body down by bending your elbows. You should lower yourself so that your upper arms are parallel to the ground. As you exhale, return to the starting position by straightening your arms. Remember; DO NOT LOCK YOUR ARMS AT THE TOP OF THIS MOVEMENT

You should complete this with a "2 second up, 2 second down tempo". This will ensure that you are getting the most out of the exercise.

Swiss ball crunches

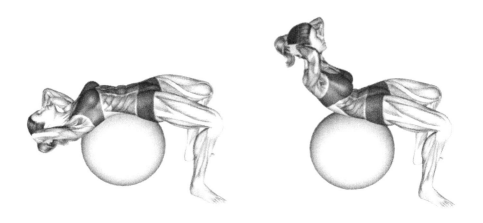

ISOLATION EXERCISE targeting: Stomach muscles (Abs)

Start position: Sit on the swiss ball with your feet flat on the ground. Walk your feet forward so the swiss ball rolls up your back and you are lying in a lying position. The swiss ball should be in your mid to lower back and you should be looking up at the sky. Place your finger tips on the side of your head.

Movement: Keeping your feet flat on the floor, you should lift your shoulder blades up, this will put immediate tension on your abdominals. You should breathe out as you do this. Your lower back should not lose contact with the swiss ball and your eyes should be in line with the sky at a 45 degree angle. Once you reach the top of the movement, lower your shoulders to the starting position and this completes one rep.

You should complete this with a "2 second up, 2 second down tempo". This will ensure that you are getting the most out of the exercise.

Pec fly

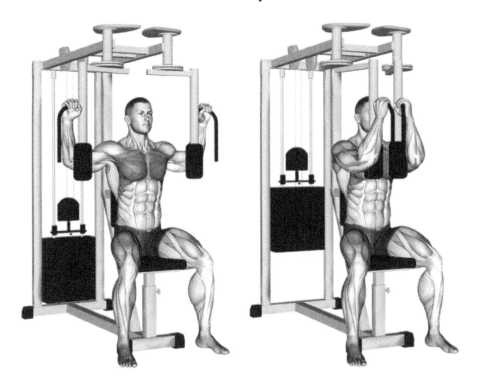

Isolation exercise targeting: Chest muscles (Pecs)

START POSITION: Adjust the seat of the machine so your arms are in line with your mid chest. Your arms should be extended out in front of you and slightly bent at the elbows after you pull each handle to your body's centreline individually. Your elbows will stay in this position throughout the exercise.

Movement: As you inhale, allow the handles to move away from your body in an arc away from your centreline. You should only let this go back to the point that you feel the stretch. This will vary from person to person. Once at this point, exhale and return to the start position.

You should complete this with a "2 second up, 2 second down tempo". This will ensure that you are getting the most out of the exercise.

Close Grip Rows

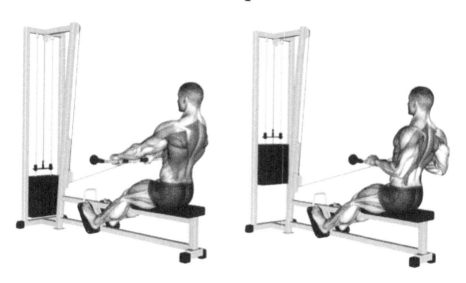

Compound exercise targeting: Back muscles (Lats)

START POSITION: Sit on the machine with your feet on the foot rests keeping your knees slightly bent back flat. Grip the handles so your hands are inside your shoulder width,you can use a "palms in grip" if you prefer. Keep your back flat and look directly forward, take the weight of the machine.

Movement: As you exhale, bring the handles towards you so that they touch your naval, your elbows should go slightly past your back. It is important that your back is kept flat. (I find that when doing rows, if I concentrate on pushing my chest forward at the top of the, movement it helps to keep my back flat). As you inhale, lower the bar back to the starting position.

You should complete this with a "2 second up, 2 second down tempo". This will ensure that you are getting the most out of the exercise.

Tricep push down on Cables

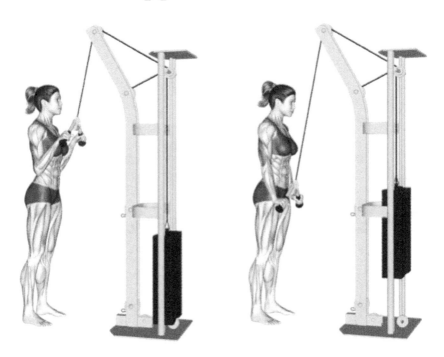

Isolation exercise targeting: Upper rear arm (Triceps)

START POSITION: Connect a rope attachment to the top setting of your cable machine. Grip the rope at the lower part of either side with your palms facing inwards. Stand with your feet shoulder width apart, toes slightly turned out, back flat and leaning forward slightly. Pull the rope down to take the weight. Your hands should be in line with your chest or there about. Your elbows should be pushed in to your body.

Movement: As you exhale, keep your elbows close to your side and push the rope down towards your quads whilst turning your palms to face the floor. At this point your palms should be nearly parallel to the floor and wrists turned up. Inhale and return to the start position. It is only the elbow joint that is moving here.

This exercise does put a lot of stress on your elbows, so if you do have week elbows, this can be done with a straight bar.

You should complete this with a "2 second up, 2 second down tempo". This will ensure that you are getting the most out of the exercise.

Lateral raises with dumbbells

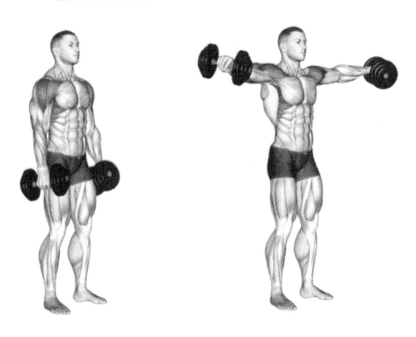

Isolation exercise targeting: Shoulder muscles (delts)

START POSITION: You can do this this sitting on a bench for a more concentrated exercise although it can be performed standing up. If you go for the bench option you should use an adjustable bench and set this so it is just under maximum upright position (1 notch back). Grab your dumbbells and sit on the bench. Allow your arms to hang down by your sides with your palms facing inwards. Keep your elbows slightly bent.

Movement: As you exhale, raise your arms so they are parallel to the ground and out to your sides. The only joint that should be moving here is your shoulder. Inhale as you lower to the start position.

You should complete this with a "2 second up, 2 second down tempo". This will ensure that you are getting the most out of the exercise.

Leg extensions

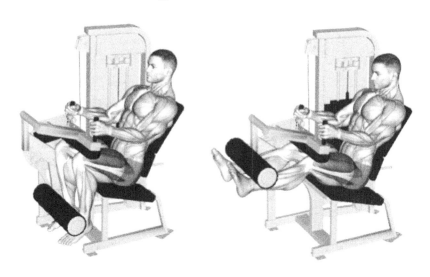

Isolation exercise targeting: Front upper leg muscles (Quads)

START POSITION: Sit on the machine and adjust so that your knees are in line with the machines hinge point. The pad should be resting on your lower shin. When your back is flat on the back rest, your hands are gripped on the machines handles or under the seat and your toes are pointed upwards (Toes should stay pointed up wards throughout the movement. This helps to target your quads more) you are ready to begin.

Movement: As you exhale, keeping your toes pointed upwards, straighten your legs, but DO NOT snap them into a locked position at the top of the movement. Once at the top of the movement, inhale and return to the start position. It is a good idea to not let the weight rest back on the stack, always keep the tension on.

You should complete this with a "2 second up, 2 second down tempo". This will ensure that you are getting the most out of the exercise.

Lying leg curl

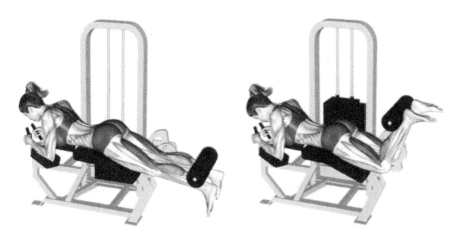

Isolation exercise targeting: Rear upper leg muscles (Hamstrings)

START POSITION: Adjust the machine so that when lying on it, you knees are in line with the hinge point. Your knees should not be in contact with the machine pad. Your quads should be resting on this. The "Working pad" should rest across your lower calf and your toes should be turned up towards your body.

Movement: As you exhale, keeping your toes pointed, bend your legs and bring the working pad up towards your glutes squeezing at the top of the movement, inhale when returning to the start position. Make sure that you fully straighten your legs when returning to the start position.

You should complete this with a "2 second up, 2 second down tempo". This will ensure that you are getting the most out of the exercise.

Calf raises

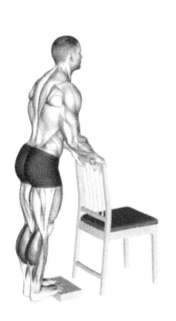 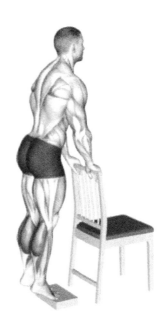

Isolation exercise targeting: Lower rear leg muscles (Calves)

START POSITION: Stand on the floor in front of the machine and adjust the height of the shoulder pads so that they are in line with your shoulders. Step onto the machine and stand with your feet hip width apart and toes facing forward. Take the weight of the working part of the machine by slowly standing up straight and grip the handles or top of the machine. (Ensure that your hands are away from any working parts)

Movement: Keep your back flat, and look to your front throughout the movement. As you exhale, raise your heels up as far as you can to feel the squeeze at the top of the movement. (I always hold this position for a second or two, to get the most out of it). As you inhale, lower your heals back down to where you feel the stretch. It is as important to get a good stretch at the bottom of the movement as the squeeze at the top. Many people neglect this factor!

You should complete this with a "2 second up, 2 second down tempo". This will ensure that you are getting the most out of the exercise.

Cable Crossover

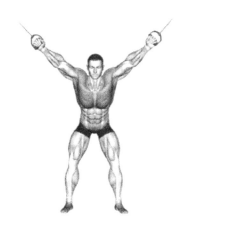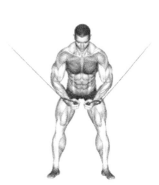

Isolation exercise targeting: Chest muscles (pecs)

START POSITION: Select the stirrup attachements for the cable machine and attach them to the high pulley. Grip these stirrups so that your palms are facing forward, your elbows should be slightly bent and locked in this position.

Movement: Keeping your elbows slightly bent, as you exhale bring your palms to meet each other at your bodys midline, rotating to finish as your little fingers on each hand connect. Once at this point return to the start position as you exhale. You should return to where you feel the stretch, this will vary from person to person.

You should complete this with a "2 second up, 2 second down tempo". This will ensure that you are getting the most out of the exercise.

Incline barbell press

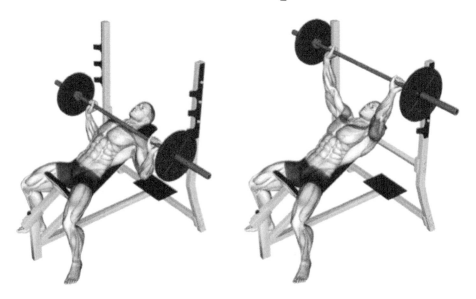

Compound exercise targeting: Upper chest muscles (Pecs)

START POSITION: Grab an adjustable bench and set it to one or two notches towards the incline position (any higher than this and you start to dilute the movement as the shoulders start to take some of the work away). Lay on the bench under a barbell on a rack or smiths machine so that your eyes are in line with the bar. Form a right angle with your arms. This will form your grip width, now grip the bar.

Movement: Lift the barbell off the rack or unhook if using a smiths machine. Straighten your arms until they are only slightly bent. As you inhale, lower the bar to your upper chest. When the bar is just about to touch, exhale as you return to the start position.

You should complete this with a "2 second up, 2 second down tempo". This will ensure that you are getting the most out of the exercise.

Concentration curls

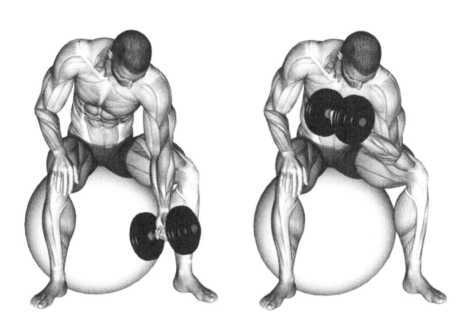

Isolation exercise targeting: Front upper arm muscles (Biceps)

START POSITION: Select a dumbbell that will allow you to perform the movement within your target rep range. You can sit on a bench, swissball or chair for this. Allow your working arm to hang down by your side with your palm facing inward. Keep your elbow slightly bent.

Movement: As you exhale, bend your elbow so your lower arm moves across your body until your palm is facing your opposite chest muscle. Return to the start position as you inhale. Remember not to lock your elbow when you return to the start position. Keep the tension on throughout the movement.

You should complete this with a "2 second up, 2 second down tempo". This will ensure that you are getting the most out of the exercise.

Stiff legged dead lifts

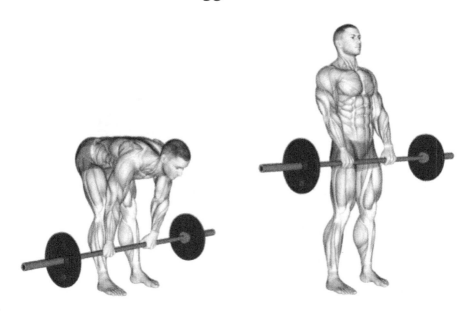

Compound exercise targeting: Rear upper leg (Hamstrings)

START POSITION: If you have a rack, it will help to place your bar on this to start with. Grip the bar with about a shoulder width gap. With your back flat and knees bent, pick your bar up so it hangs just in front of your quads. Ensure that your feet are hip width apart and are facing forward.

Movement: You do not need to keep your legs locked in a straight position. Keep your knees slightly bent and with a flat back and arms slightly bent at the elbows, exhale as you lower the weight forward, bending at your hips. You should lower the bar to the point that you feel the stretch. This will vary from person to person. Inhale as you slowly return to the start position whilst maintaining a flat back and slightly bent knees.

You may need to stand on a step whilst doing this movement to allow the weight some ground clearance.

You should complete this with a "3 second up, 3 second down tempo". This will ensure that you are getting the most out of the exercise.

Lateral cable raises

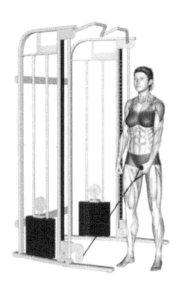 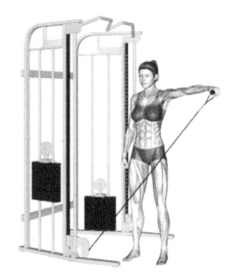

Isolation exercise targeting: Shoulder muscles (Delts)

START POSITION: Select a stirrup attachment and hook this to the bottom setting of your cable machine. Stand with the pulley system to one side and pick up the stirrup with the opposite hand. Allow your working arm to hang down by your side with your palm facing inwards. Keep your elbow slightly bent.

Movement: As you exhale, raise your arm so it is parallel to the ground and out to your side. The only joint that should be moving here is your shoulder. Inhale as you lower to the start position. Do not let the weight rest back on the stack. Keep the tension on throughout the movement.

You should complete this with a "2 second up, 2 second down tempo". This will ensure that you are getting the most out of the exercise.

Bent over dumbbell raises

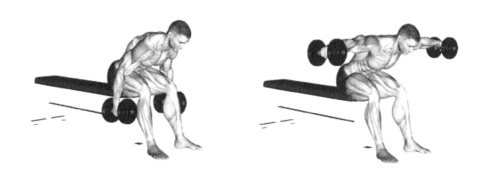

Isolation exercise targeting: Rear shoulder muscles (Read delts)

START POSITION: Grab an adjustable bench and set it so it is in a flat position. Select your dumbbells and sit on the bench placing the dumbbells on the floor underneath your hamstrings. Extend your feet out in front of you slightly, keeping them flat on the floor. Keeping your glutes in contact with the bench, bring your chest to meet your knees. Pick up the dumbbells with your palms facing inwards and bend your elbows slightly.

Movement: As you exhale, keeping your elbows slightly bent but locked in this position raise your arms upward so that your palms are parallel to the floor whilst squeezing your shoulder blades together. Inhale as you return to the start position.

(I always do these facing a mirror and keep my head up so I can see my form. It is very tempting to cheat on these. If you don't glance every once in a while you may not even notice that you are sitting up more and more on each rep)

You should complete this with a "2 second up, 2 second down tempo". This will ensure that you are getting the most out of the exercise.

Barbell squats

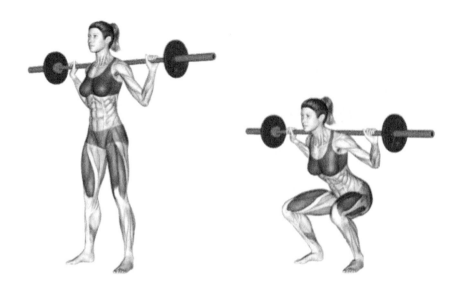

Compound exercise targeting: Leg muscles

START POSITION: Stand with your feet hip-width apart, toes slightly turned out. The bar should be resting across your shoulders and traps. Grip the bar, palms facing forward and at spacing that is comfortable. Pick a point on a wall or in the distance that is eye level or higher and look at this throughout the movement. This will help you keep your posture and maintain correct form.

Movement: Keeping your feet flat on the floor, as you breathe in, bend your knees until your quads (Upper legs) are parallel to the ground. Push back through your heels to starting position. Whilst breathing out. Ensure that you are always looking straight ahead or slightly up. This will help you keep good posture. This completes one rep.

Shrugs

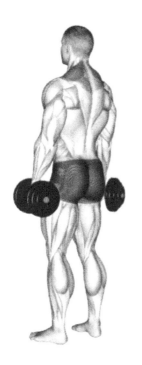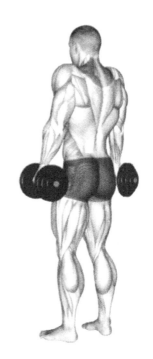

Isolation exercise targeting: Upper shoulder (Traps)

START POSITION: Select a barbell or a set of dumbbells and place on a rack (if you have one, this just helps with the starting position but is not essential.). Grip the bar about shoulder width apart. Stand with your feet hip width apart and toes slightly turned out. Pick up the weights so they rests just in front of your quads (for a barbell) or just on your outer quads (for dumbbells). Your elbows should be slightly bent throughout the movement.

Movement: As you exhale, keep your elbows as they are and lift your shoulders up towards your ears. You can get a good squeeze here if you have the right weight. Inhale as you return to the start position. (Many people will overload the bar for some reason on this exercise and therefore dilute the exercise a lot. A good tip is to start with a light weight and feel the muscle working correctly. You will get way better results)

You should complete this with a "2 second up, 2 second down tempo". This will ensure that you are getting the most out of the exercise.

Preparing for a competition

Prepping for a stage show or contest can be tough. If you decide to take on this challenge, you will want to be at your best on the day of the show. It is important to know that there is no "ultimate way" to prep as everyone who wants to embark on this task will be different. Everyone will have a different journey, diet and their own set of challenges.

But I would like to outline some factors that will most likely be the same for all who decide to up their game and take on this challenging task.

Contest prep is a whole other subject and I just plan to scratch the surface in this section and give you a heads up on what to expect.

There are millions of people that are involved in bodybuilding in some way or another. The majority of these people will never take the next step and actually train, diet and don posing trunks for a stage show or competition.

The more that your physique develops as you make progress on your bodybuilding journey, the more likely it is that you would like to try a competition. As you may know already, bodybuilding is a lifestyle more than it is a hobby.

It is hard to build your body up and this process requires a lot of consistency and effort. Changing your body shape by visiting the gym, on a regular basis is one thing but getting yourself ready for a competition is taking this to a whole new level.

For most people who have developed a strong muscular foundation, it will require around twenty weeks of extreme dedication prior to the show. Believe it or not most of the work to get ready is done out of the gym!

First and foremost, your diet needs to be right. This is by far the toughest part. To get a really freaky condition, you need to cut out most foods that you would normally eat and a huge amount that are actually deemed as healthy.

For the most part, your diet will be the same every single day, it will be fairly bland as you are very limited on flavourings that you can use on your food.

You will have to get used to cooking a lot of food every day and by that I mean EVERY day. There can be no excuses for missing any one of your six, eight or even ten meals.

With a lot of cooking comes a lot of washing up so you really need to stay on top of this. You have to be organised when it comes to pre contest prep.

You will need to get up earlier to do your cardio before work and you will need to go to bed later in order to prepare your food and get your final meal in.

Before you start, make sure that you have plenty of money saved up. You will probably be eating as much as a family of four!

Food and supplements are a huge expense at this point. If you can buy at wholesale, it will cut the cost down a fair bit.

As well as keeping your diet sharp, you will also have to throw in more cardio and posing sessions. You have to learn to pose and pose well. You could have the best physique on stage, but if the judges can't see it, they can't judge it.

Posing is hard work! If you have never done this before, you may think it looks easy to stand there and flex a few muscles for 30 minutes or so. Go and see a posing coach and you will probably change your mind.

Your social life will suffer. You will find it harder to go to events, parties and out for meals as you will have to make sure that you bring your food with you and also make sure you can eat it at the time that it needs to be eaten.

Your family life will change. The best that you can hope for is the support from your friends and family. These guys will be on the journey with you and they will share in your triumph when you hold your trophy and stand on the winner's podium.

Some of this may sound negative but this is what it's all about. If you do decide to take up the challenge, you will have a better chance of seeing it through if you know what to expect.

It is probably fair to say that most spectators of the sport do not understand the dedication, hardship and determination that these guys on stage have put themselves through to get to where they are.

If you are going to take up this challenge and give it a go for the first time, other than understanding what is required of you, you should also not try to do this by yourself. You should seek advice from someone who has done this before successfully.

Getting yourself ready for a bodybuilding show is very hard. There are a lot of things that you have to be aware of. If you have a mentor, you will pick up tips and tricks that you won't have heard of before. If your mentor has been successful in the past, listen to them! Do what they say and do not try to do your own thing.

I hope that this has given you a small insight into competition preparation and I hope that you decide to go ahead with it. To stand onstage knowing the amount of effort that you have put in to get there in front of an admirable crowd is a great feeling. And to pick up a trophy is even better! Your struggle is more than rewarded when you stand under those bright lights looking tanned and sculpted.

"It's all worth it"

Conclusion

So this was your year of bodybuilding. Once that you complete the full years training I suggest that you reassess yourself.

You may find that you have a weak muscle group. In this case you should maybe add another exercise for this muscle group and/ or drop an exercise for one of your more developed muscle groups.

If you have had well balanced development, you can just start again from week 1. Your body will still develop and you may find that you are lifting more weight on all of the exercises.

This is by no means the "definitive bodybuilding programme". There is no such thing. This is a guide that uses progressive training techniques.

By training in this way, you will ensure that your muscles are constantly being stressed enough to cause continued muscle growth.

Bodybuilding is a way of life. If you are disciplined, consistent, you make your training sessions count, and you realise that it will take time for your muscles to develop, you will get good results.

You need to be disciplined; it is all too easy to say:

"I've had a hard day at work, Il give my training a miss today"

Or

"I'm going to skip this meal, Il pick up something a bit more tasty later on"

The thing is, as soon as you start missing training sessions or eating junk food , it will become easier to miss another session or eat even more junk food.

Plan your rest days and cheat meals and stick to them.

You need to be consistent. It's no good training for a week or two and then having a week off. You need to train and eat consistently to earn and keep your new muscle. If you are happy with 20% of the results, put in 20% of the work.

Even when you are tired or if you have had a bad day, you should still give 100% when you are in the gym. Make sure that you make every rep of every set count.

It's one thing going to the gym and "Going through the motions", it's another thing going to the gym and busting your balls.

Don't go through the motions! Go to the gym and make your workouts count.

With successful bodybuilding, comes great strength of character and you will develop some great "tools" that you can use in other areas of your life. You will also learn a lot about yourself and what you are capable of achieving.

If you work on this way of thinking, you are well on your way to building yourself a great body and mind. Don't be the guy or gal who just "talks the talk". Get yourself prepared, plan out your year of bodybuilding correctly and walk the walk of a bodybuilder!

"There are no excuses! If you really want to earn a bodybuilders physique, go out and earn it!"

Good luck! I wish you all the best in your efforts. I would love to hear how you get on with this.

Connect with Jim

VISIT MY BLOG AT www.jimshealthandmuscle.com[1] for healthy recipes, training ideas and more

Don't forget to drop by and "Like" my facebook page atwww.facebook.com/JimsHealthAndMuscle[2]or follow me on twitter @jimshm[3]

---

1. http://www.jimshealthandmuscle.com

2. http://www.facebook.com/JimsHealthAndMuscle

3. https://twitter.com/jimsHM

Made in the USA
Monee, IL
28 December 2022

23659574R00066